MW00975179

For my l'il sis Ang

The closest thing any person will ever get to being a flower faery; because she thirsts for knowledge.

Beauty is a fragile gift.

Ovid

Introduction

I grew up surrounded by essential oils and pots of creams. My mom, Jill Bruce, ran (still runs, I should say) one of the first aromatherapy manufacturing companies in the world. Over the years, she has treated hundreds of thousands of people with aches and pains and poorly skins. Training with her was a gift.

If you looked at her skin you would say she was twenty years younger, and actually, now, I think she finds it a bit of a curse. I suspect she silently envies those people who enjoy allowances for being old! She would love more people to give up their seats on the bus for her. After all she is nearly 70!

Mom is passionate about skin care. I have to admit, I am not! I kinda take my skin for granted and slap on some oils and that is that. Luckily for me, my complexion does not give me away very often. I learned skin care from the Master Apothecary. Mom's creams are sublime beyond compare. I have built my own sets of tricks of the trade upon the strong foundation she gave me.

The first thing to know is that skin care is never only about the skin. A million other things affect it, diet, hormones, even the environment where you work. Genetics plays a very big part too, from the beautiful skin I inherited from my mother, to the familial likelihood of developing eczema.

The second thing to remember is aromatherapy is a sensual art. That is: we use every one of our senses to discern which oils will become the elixir for a person's skin. In this book, not only will I show you how to make your own creams, toners and masques from scratch, but I'll show you how to listen with your eyes and hear through your fingers! A good therapist employs all of their five senses and utilises their sixth one too. Here, in this book, we open a portal to heal really sad skin in its worst possible state and take it, quickly and easily, into a smooth and beautifully radiant condition.

I have been careful to design this book in a way that prevents the sensation of being completely overwhelmed that I feel some books can create. I am permanently frustrated with kindle books, when I look at the recipes and think "I haven't got any of these oils" and *I* have 450 bottles of the flipping things, so goodness knows what a newcomer must feel!

Here, I have identified the definitive oils for treating dry skin and built around those. There are some expensive ones, rose, jasmine, neroli and violet leaf, for instance...but I also show you how to get around using those too. They are the best...but not the *only* choices. In fact, if you don't even have a single bottle of essential oil, that's OK too. I show you how to make a start on improving your skin simply working with fresh fruit you'll have in the kitchen.

So come on, step in side...I'll show you what treats exist in my bathroom (it's freshly tiled you know!) and I'll show you how to create a whole new face for you to smile out from.

Table of Contents

The skill of creating really good skin care is to design it entirely around the individual you have in mind. That is probably you, but it might not be. I have created this book in a way to make it very simple for you to make a batch of Christmas presents for friends, too, for instance.

If you simply rush for a bottle of frankincense, it will help wrinkles and prevent dryness far better than your main stream boutique face creams but it is not bespoke. It addresses how dehydrated the skin has become, but nothing more. Blackheads, open pores and broken capillaries, for example, still remain. The skin looks better, good even, perhaps. But you still couldn't describe it as radiant.

Here, we are looking at the difference between high end High Street and then the kind of Saville Row tailoring in a suit you'd see David Beckham wearing. Judging from the number of likes a picture of David's "watch" got on my Facebook page, I think we all appreciate when something fits perfectly! (Just in case any of you did not see it...and for those of you who did...it would be rude not to I think... https://pbs.twimg.com/media/CE309LQXIAAbaed.jpg:large)

So here, in the book, I aim to teach you how to embroider absolutely as much detail as you possibly can into blends. The objective is to have your complexion singing anthems of hurrah in celebrations of the oils you have chosen.

The easiest way to do this is to look at it in stages moving deeper and deeper into the skin. By the end of the book you will not only be able to make creams to feed your skin back to health, but you will understand what has happened to make it that way in the first place and have the confidence to create your very own skin care solutions. I'll hold your hand, but by the end you will be free-wheeling, stabilisers off. You will be able to improve anyone's skin with just a couple of bottles of essential oils coupled with bucketfuls of knowhow.

Clearly making a cream for your *own* skin is going to be easier than making one for someone else's. You have intimate knowledge of how *your* skin reacts in certain weathers, but other people's...that's not to so easy. And actually it can be a pretty delicate topic to address really, can't it?

So I have added some twists and turns into the book that will have your friends wondering if you have taken up scrying in some kind of crystal ball. How else could you have gained such an understanding of the skin which *they* thought appeared flawless to the rest of the world? It might just *be* immaculate under their foundation; but I promise you, you can rely on aromatherapy to make it *even* better.

To understand skin care really well, you first need to understand what each bit does in the job, I think.

The Anatomy of the skin

Don't skip this section...I know, I would too, but don't. Treating the skin is far less bewildering when you have an understanding of what it is and what it does, but most of all, how it does it.

The first thing to grasp is that the skin is an organ. In fact, it is the largest organ in the body. It has many jobs to do. These are:

- It holds the organs in place and it also maintains fat and water levels inside of the body
- In protects us from outside infections and microbes
- It regulates body temperature from extreme heat or cold.
- It manufactures vitamin D in sunlight. This vitamin D is very important because not only does it support healthy teeth and bones but it is also has a part to play in regulating mood and also guarding against some autoimmune conditions.

It is formed of *epithelial tissue*. This means it is a tissue that is just one single layer of tissue thick. In some places of the body this will be delicate and thin...on the lips for instance, but in others it needs to be robust and hard and so many layers accumulate as they would on the heels of the feet, for instance.

The anatomy of the organ is complex and it is made up of many layers of cells.

Fundamentally though, it can be broken down into three main layers.

- The epidermis
- The dermis
- The subcutaneous layer

Let's look at each layer in turn.

Epidermis

This is the outermost layer of the skin, the bit you can see and feel and actually, this too, can be divided into its own two layers. The top most part is called the **Stratum Corneum** (Often it is also referred to as the horny layer).

This layer is composed entirely of **dead cells.** *Millions and millions* of dead cells. Give your arm a brisk rub and the chances are you will see some fall free into the air. When you get wet in the bath, these will easily peel away. Remember that. This is useful to utilise later on.

So where have these come from? Well, they have been pushed up from layer just beneath. We call this the **granular layer**.

This "region" acts almost like a nursery for cells called keratinocytes formed on the *basal layer* below. Here, new cells strengthen and mature, ready for their rise to the stratum corneum. They flatten and die here, as they rise through. Where previously the cell had a nucleus to instruct the cell to divide, a protein, keratin, forms to take its place.

Keratin is hard and durable so water struggles to get through it. This is how skin is *virtually* waterproof and is able to protect the body from any invasive bacteria etc.

This layer also contains melanocytes which form the melanin pigment which (amongst other functions) changes the skin colour as we tan in sunlight. Providing the body has enough vitamins and minerals present, just 10 minutes a day in sunlight with make enough vitamin D for the body's needs.

At the very base of the epidermis we find the germinative or basal layer. The cells of the basal layer continuously divide and transform into keratinocytes. This continual cycle means that the cells in the stratum layer are always readily replaced. Remember that term **keratinocytes**...it will be very useful later.

So, let's imagine the life cycle of the cell. It is formed in the granular (or basal) layer, it sits for a while in the middle layer where it grows and fattens up. It dies and flattens out, filling with protein and toughening up. Then it is pushed up by even newer cells that want to access the feeding frenzy. It goes up the top layer and eventually, about a month after it was first formed, it will flake away.

Well....that's the plan anyway. We'll come back to that in a moment.

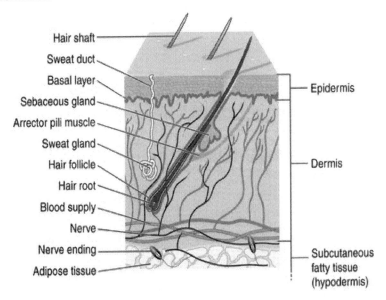

The epidermis itself has no blood supply, but the base of the germinative layer is wav,y allowing plenty of blood supply to skin. These blood vessels keep the skin vital with its supply of nourishment. If there is poor circulation, then inevitably nutrients are compromised and this will eventually affect the skin's health.

The dermis contains blood vessels, sweat glands, hair follicles and sebaceous glands. These are all surrounded by the connective tissue which helps with the skin's elasticity.

The tiny blood vessels within the skin are called **capillaries.** They curl around into tiny branches and loops as they get closer to the surface of the skin and control the body's temperature. They expand and open up when warm so they can allow heat to escape. Conversely, when it is cold, they will shrink, causing the rosy appearance of heat and cold fingers in the snow. Sweat glands also play a large part in keeping the body's temperature even.

Every hair on the body grows out of a duct called the hair follicle. The part of the hair you can see is dead and is made up mainly from keratin. In each follicle is a tiny muscle called the **hair erector muscle** which literally makes our hair stand up on end; in much earlier incarnations of man, these would have allowed the hairs over the body to fluff up and keep our cave forefathers warm.

Subcutaneous fat also plays a part in keeping people warm. Eskimos have developed thicker pads of this fat over their eyes which tend to be exposed to the cold. This subcutaneous fat is the reason why plumper people tend to have younger looking, unlined complexions and those who have been on crash diets may develop saggy faces.

Dysfunction of the skin

Oxidation

Oxidation is what causes cells to age and eventually die. It is at the root of diseases such as cancers and tumours, the breaking down of the lungs in conditions such as COPD and a whole host of other delights, including aging our skin. This oxidation is caused by something called *free radicals.*

To understand these, the first thing you need to comprehend is the smallest particle, an atom, either has a positive or negative charge. Here we are interested in **electrons which are negatively charged.**

Free radicals are atoms or groups of atoms with an odd (unpaired) number of electrons. These are formed when oxygen interacts with certain molecules. Radicals are very, very reactive and they tend to set off chain reactions. Most importantly these negatively interact with the cell membrane and other components of the cells such as your DNA. As the radicals interfere with the cells, they oxidise, decay and break down...and then we see the chain reaction spread like wildfire through the cells.

We can't stop it. It is a natural process.

We can slow it down.

The first and most important thing to say is please stop smoking if you are. Smoking is the single biggest contributor to oxidation in your body. It affects your skin badly, but now think of what it is doing to your insides.

You will have heard of the best weapon we have against free radicals. **These are anti-oxidants.**

Antioxidants interact safely with free radicals. They abort the chain reaction before any of the vital molecules are damaged. There are enzyme systems existing naturally in the body that scavenge free radicals, but principally we should try to get these from diet. (Hence the need for so many fruits and vegetables in a day.)

The main vitamin antioxidants are **vitamin E, beta-carotene, and vitamin C** as well as a trace metal, **selenium.**

Throughout the book we will meet anti-oxidant ingredients. Every time you do, smile gleefully and pop it onto your shopping list. Essential oils will improve your skin, anti-oxidants will slow down your body's (and thus your skin's) physical aging.

Sebaceous Glands

In skin care, the **sebaceous glands** are probably the most important component. The number of sebaceous glands varies around the body. On the nose and chin, for example, there are far more than the elbows and knees. These small glands open up into the hair follicle and secrete an oily substance called **sebum.** This covers the skin with a thin film of oil. Fresh sebum is extremely antiseptic so it protects the body from bacteria. Problems only start to arise when the balance in the sebum slides out of kilter. Too much sebum and we begin to struggle with greasy hair and skin. Too little and the skin becomes dry and brittle.

Flaking Skin

Now, try to imagine skin cells as bricks in a very large structure. For a while these bricks could support their own weight but as the structure gets bigger, these bricks would need to be held together by iron rods to strengthen the support. In your skin, these iron rods are binders called *corneodesmosomes*. The mortar holding the bricks together, is comprised of molecules containing waxes and fats called **lipids**.

Consider then, with skin problems such as eczema or dry skin, the skin barrier is thinner than it would normally be. These iron rods no longer have adequate protection from external forces at work. It's a bit like the roof is off the construction now and so these iron rods are cast open to the elements. With no barrier covering, they deteriorate and eventually they snap. Now in dry skin complaints and particularly in eczema, this is exactly what happens. The corneodesmosomes snap too early causing this flaking of the skin that we see. Their skin cell cycle is far shorter than the month we would hope to see and it means they always have this troubling dry flaky skin.

Emotions and the Skin

The skin betrays more about what were feeling in our hearts than any other organ, not least because it is the only one on display! Bizarrely, the correlating emotions to do with the skin are exactly that...they convey how we feel about the way we perceive that the world sees us.

If you look like s**t, ask yourself how you feel about the way you behaved last night, or about what is going on in life in general. If you are all loved up and happy, your skin will glow along with you. When it all starts to crumble, so you will see your skin care regime needs to move up a notch too. Here, in this book there is no need to delve deeply into the psychology of the skin, but for those who have deeper concerns you will find my book The Aromatherapy Eczema Treatment very helpful, I think.

Ayurvedic Aromatherapy

An Apology...

As we enter into the recipes etc. now, I had better warn you: you are going to hate my spelling in this book if you are American. I acquiesced on the cover (moisturizer!), but I am afraid writing all these US spellings really jars with me. I worked hard on my spelling tests at school and so....

You are stuck with moisturiser, colour and favourite amongst others spellings, sadly. The English readers will be dancing a jig right now, I am sure! The rest of you, please try not to hyperventilate and twitch in annoyance too much, please. Frowning at my spelling will only give you wrinkles....

Next, I am going to take it as read that you will have downloaded your free book *The Complete Guide to Clinical Aromatherapy and The Essential Oils of The Physical Body*, and shall not cover old ground about what essential oils are and how to use them. If you haven't, it is 300 pages of learning that will improve your skills. <u>Download it now.</u>

Ayurvedic Aromatherapy

I think it would be fair to suggest when aromatherapy started to gather momentum in the 1960s it would have taken on many of the principles of Ayurveda, not least that of the subtle bodies.

Regarded as the mother of medicine, Ayurvedic writings date back five thousand years. Written in Sanskrit, the ancient teachings of the Vedas speak of a person in terms of three elements. The *outer body*, which we would know as skin, hair, teeth; the things we as a Western world would name as indicators for beauty. Then they have the *inner body,* which is bones, internal processes such as digestion etc, but also thoughts and ideas too. When the inner and outer body are in harmony then their third element, the *shining aspect*, radiates through.

Essentially it is the mind, body spirit concept worded in a different way. I actually think it makes for easier understanding for the person who struggles to grasp the idea of their spirituality.

This is a massive realm, that I am sure is many books in its own right, but I am including it because I find it is a very useful way of making clever guesses about what people might be struggling with under the surface...or actually their lipstick and foundation!!!

If you want to make a gift for someone and you don't want to make a risky choice about their skin then Ayurveda is very good at grouping people so you can make an educated gamble. It should also help you to discern how, changing some things you are eating will probably improve your skin dryness no end.

What's more of all the ancient medicines Ayurveda provides the biggest emphasis on beauty and so its wisdom is both arcane and sacrosanct. Most of the essential oils we use, particularly for dry skin, in aromatherapy can be traced back to plants in their skin care usage through Ayurveda for about five millennia.

Their teachings say that in the very centre of perfection is nothing, and yet it is made up of everything.

What?

Yes, I did the same. This helped me.

Consider white light. It appears as the whiteness of nothing, but if you shine it through a prism (or a raindrop for example) it disturbs the rays and you are able to see many colours; in fact, there is every colour of the rainbow.

Everything in life is comprised of one of five elements: Air, Water, Fire, Earth, Ether (or space). In fact, every element in the universe is found in the human body. Disturbance then, shatters the elements into groups and we call these the doshas. **In Ayurveda you are always aiming to reduce the excess of** your dosha to bring it into harmony with the rest of the group....to nothingness.

So it follows then, that we should be able to heal an imbalance by using something else natural to bring the body into that alignment. Ayurveda uses herbs and spices, foods generally and *essential oils.*

At the moment you were conceived your dosha was determined. This is called your *pakruti.* The three dosha are vata, pitta and kapha. Very few people are entirely one dosha, more likely two or even a mix of all three, but usually we are able to see a predominant trend. Whilst pakruti never completely changes, it does fluctuate with emotions, with the seasons and even times of the day. Mostly though, it is affected by diet. When there is an imbalance, we call this *vikruti.*

The Doshas

Vata –Earth and Air
The Vata is dosha attributed to movement. People of this pakruti share many qualities with their specific season of autumn. They are light, mobile, dry, brittle. Vata people are very restless. They are creative and can almost be a little flighty. They will often have dry skin. Of all the doshas they suffer from constitution the most. They also find it difficult to

settle and concentrate, in particular they struggle to sleep. They have more energy in the morning and can be verging on hyper at night.

As we age, naturally become more vata. The skin gets drier, we become more forgetful, have less stamina, think more but act less, our bones become more brittle....

Physiologically they are tall, slender, flat chested (or actually sometimes disproportionately large chested). They have long limbs especially fingers and can often struggle to look or even be coordinated.

Vatas are naughty eaters. In that they don't. They skip meals or even forget to have them. Consequently their immune is low, naturally they are very prone to chills and this makes it even harder for them to concentrate

Vata people are seldom troubled by having to lose weight, by contrast, gaining it is their problem. Because they are frenetic by nature and tend not to eat enough either, there is rarely fat on their bones.

If you know someone who is what I would call a flibbety gibbet, very restless, thinks very quickly (and is more theories than action) then it is likely they will be a vata and thus have drier skin. Likewise they will have those gorgeous athletic bodies and very long limbs and fingers. Does this help you at all?

Pitta- Fire and Water

Pitta is summer. It is hot and sweaty and excited! I'm a pitta, and if the lustrous red locks weren't out of a bottle they would perhaps have given it away. My very freckly, pale complexion certainly does. Pittas are fiery, they are driven and ambitious and they are sharp. For that read either intellectually or nasty with their words; both would be true. As I said, they tend to have red, blonde or silver grey hair, warm but pale skin, often covered in freckles.

For pitta read *sensitive*; whether that means hot and sensitive skin, moody by nature, temperamental or even in constitution. There is only one thing which is not sensitive in a pitta...and that's his belly. A pitta, eats, eats and eats some more. They like to eat socially and if a pitta person misses their lunch, you had better get out of their way

Kapha –Earth and Water

For kapha read *unmovable*. By nature these are life's lovely plodders. Nothing fazes them. They are so chilled; always got a smile on their faces. They have lustrous cream skin, and massive big white teeth. Their faces have lovely exotic large features, in particular their gorgeously full lips. Everything about a kapha is large, it's heavy and it is usually slow.

So on the good side, these people go with the flow, on the down side, you will often feel like you want to put a rocket under them. Kaphas don't like change and so like everything else in their lives, the changes through treatment will probably be slow too. On the upside it is usually easy to see what caused their issues in the first place...new software at work, or new boss, moving house, even kids going away to uni. If it involves change, they will find it hard.

This implies they are lazy, and it is true they do like their beds but....Of all the doshas kapha have stamina. They will work way into the night and will always see a project through to the very end. And of course with their size and stamina they have immense strength. For an employer they are a godsend because they are such a reliable set of hands.

Problems, as you might imagine, for kapha dosha are congestion, water retention, constipation, puffy eyes and ankles; anything to do with accumulation or a traffic jam effect.

As I said, not many people are all one dosha, and similarly there are very few who are tridoshic, all three equally. Most people find they have elements of two, with one more than the other. I am Pitta - Kapha, and my husband is Kapha Pitta. This means that he and I understand each other very well but he and my son, who is vata-kapha are continuously at odds. The boy is all theory and all up in his head, the man is practical application and diligence all of the way. Both are incredible grafters but in entirely differing ways.

By eating foods which irritate our tissues we can over or under stimulate them. Pitta gets hotter, sharper and burnt out! Often this leads to sensitivity means rashes etc. (hello eczema, rosacea and sensitive skins!), vata gets even more hyper, drier and colder, and kapha gets ever more cynical, slow and also cold. You will also see their skins become oilier.

Agni is the digestive fire. In Ayurveda it is believed that **all healing stems from the digestive system**. It must be clean of toxins and also be nurtured in a way that agni can burn vigorously and long.

Ama
If agni is too sluggish to process foods or it burns too hot then toxicity is produced and we call this ama. Ama enters the blood system and then is taken to every tissue in the body. So then it pervades very quickly bringing dis-ease and dis-order.

If you can identify which is the predominant pitta you are treating it will help you chose foods and oils to heal the body *quicker*.

Anti Doshic Diet

For those of you who are interested in the changes Ayurveda can bring, I'll give a swift outline of who should eat what.

Vata Foods

You will remember these are people, not only with dry skin but who are also the most restless of people. By nature they feel the cold and suffer from dryness generally. (Incidentally we can say dryness of the mouth, vaginal dryness, not sweating very much...) so we aim for food which is warm, moist, sweet or salty for their best foods.

For example, we would always want a vata to cook their food. Their constitution is too delicate to break down tough enzymes from raw. They should choose fruits which are heavy and raise blood sugar like avocado, banana and papaya. A raw diet will only serve to make them more vata.

When choosing vegetables they should look for warming roots like squash and beetroot and carrot. They should avoid very leafy green veg like cabbage or kale because it simply makes them to gassy.

Vatas don't do very well with legumes, again because of the gas, so they should opt for smaller versions like lentils and definitely step away larger varieties such as pinto and kidney.

Grains work very well with the vata constitution because they are so warming and often they do best by moistening them by stirring through butter or some oil.

Fish is their best choice of protein, but they also do well on organic white meats.

Pitta

Because of their fiery and sharp disposition we are looking for foods which will calm, cool and sooth. Tropical fruits do this very well, especially coconut. They do very well on brassica group of foods, so sprouts, cabbage and broccoli are all up there. They should look for cooling foods such as squash, cucumber as their primary foods, and avoid more acidic tomatoes and red peppers.

Beans, beans and more beans for pitta. They are filling, an excellent source of protein and they do not carry fat.

The sweet grains are lovely for pitta, choose jasmine or basmati. Pitta should minimise red meat and eggs. White meats are fine but the saltiness of sea food is too much, choose river fishes like salmon and trout.

Kaphas

These do best on a vegetarian diet really, since it is far less heavy. However they should opt for dry foods, hot and spicy foods and bitter and stringent choices. Clearly oily would be too fattening and moist foods would make the "mud" element even heavier.

They should avoid fruits which are high in sugar like banana and avocados. Opt for sour versions of apples, pears and cranberries, for instance.

All vegetables are good really but they should restrict the heavier root vegetables like beets and swedes.

Of all the vegetables, the heavy leafy greens work best, so cabbage, sprouts and kale.

Again for kaphas, beans make a great choice.

Grains can be problematic for kapha because their starchiness only further slows them down. Good choices include oats, rye and quinoa.

White meat works well with this constitution if they choose not to go vegetarian. They should also try to limit dairy because it can add to mucous build up in their system.

Now as a pitta I suppose I should be naturally drawn the foods which are good for me, but to my eye, I think pittas come off best. To me the kapha diet does not bear thinking about, it's almost as if they can have nothing. So....everything in moderation people, encourage this eating as a pointer but probably not the rule.

Oils to reduce vata

Remember we are looking to soothe, slow and warm.

Neroli, lemon, geranium, basil, cypress, geranium, angelica, basic, carrot, costus, cumin, fennel, frankincense, ginger, jasmine, orange, patchouli, tarragon, vetiver, ylang ylang

Oils to reduce pitta

In this group we are aiming to reduce sensitivity, cool and chill.

Rose, sandalwood, mint, sweet orange, jasmine, ylang ylang, lavender, in particular alpine or highland lavender, grapefruit, sweet orange, german chamomile, coriander, melissa and spikenard.

Oils to reduce kapha

This is the group of oils to invigorate and stimulate

Juniper, eucalyptus, camphor, clove, lavender, rosemary, eucalyptus, marjoram, melissa, lemon, peppermint, black pepper, clary sage clove, silver fir, helichrysm, lemon, rosemary, black spruce tea tree, lemon verbena

To put it into the most basic of contexts: If you wanted to relax a pitta person you might choose Rose, orange, and spikenard, to help them to chill. But if you wanted to have the same effects for a vata you might decide to go for Neroli, patchouli and ginger to warm and cosy them.

The Skin and Vitamins

We have already seen that the skin is an organ and as such it needs fuel. The main nutrients which provide these are vitamins which are absorbed from food, through the small intestine and are then distributed around the body via the blood, but...

We can add these into the mix by putting them into creams, too. Now, **essential oils** themselves **do not contain vitamins,** but **carrier oils do.** If you have not already downloaded my permafree book The Complete Guide to Clinical Aromatherapy and The Eseential Oils of the Physical Body, I would urge you to do so because there is a great more specific information about essential oils included in there. So, I have created a short list of the main beneficial vitamins for skin and the carrier oils (and nut butters if appropriate) for you to add into your mix should you want to later.

Vitamin A
Helps guard against:

- Wrinkles
- Smoothes wrinkles and fine lines
- Fades brown spots

Find it in:

Apricot kernel, Almond, Carrot, Kukui nut, Rosehip oils

Sunlight deactivates retinol in Vitamin A so it is important that this **is only used in a night cream**. Put it on before you go to bed so it can work with your body's regenerative processes.

Vitamin B 3

- Reduces redness
- Increases production of ceramides and fatty acids. This gives the skin a much more powerful barrier to trap and retain moisturiser better. This very good if the skin is very dry or sensitive and will also reduce areas of increased dark spots

Find B3 in *groundnut (peanut), sesame, sunflower and avocado* oils

Vitamin C

- Spots
- Vitamin C scavenges free radicals that oxidise cells and cause wrinkles and sagging.
- It fades brown spots, fine lines and discolouration.

Find Vitamin C in *Kukui nut and Rosehip oils*

Vitamin E

- Vitamin E neutralises free radicals.
- Research shows that if you can use it *before exposure to sunlight* it reduces dryness and redness.

Find vitamin E in *Almond, Avocado, Boabub, Carrot, Coconut, Jojoba, Soy and Wheatgerm oils.*

Vitamin K

- Reduces redness
- Protects against broken capillaries
- Reduces Dark circles under the eyes

Find it in *Canola (Rapeseed) and Olive oils*

Basic Skin Types

I am deliberately keeping the number of oils I use small in this book. One of my pet hates is buying a book and thinking I cannot afford to buy all the different components to make something. These are the quintessential oils for dry skin. As you build your set you will become more and more adept at finding other things to do with them outside of skin care. I would be doing myself a disservice if I did not point out that I have written whole books about Rose and Vetiver for instance. They are wondrous for the skin, but there are many other things you can do with them, either following the lines of modern medicinal studies or in ways that the ancients have used them before.

Cleopatra was a big fan of Rose and of Neroli. Both are exquisite oils for dry skin. Neroli is better for more mature skins and for those that have become toughened by the weather or by smoking. Use either rose otto essential oil or rose absolute. Both are sublime, although the absolute is probably richer and gives as gorgeous honey glow to the cream.

Remember I mentioned keratinocytes in the anatomy? Well, scientific research has now proven that rose *absolute* feeds these cells, making the new cells formed much stronger and healthier. For this reason, and the fact that I love it, rose absolute is always going to be my own personal choice for skin care. If you have otto though, it is still superlative...simply, not yet *proven* to work in the same way.

Neroli, for those of you who don't know, is orange blossom and is available as an essential oil.

There are receipts from Napoleon's personal perfumer that show Josephine adored Jasmine (although it is said Napoleon would order her not to bathe for when he came back from battle as he adored her scent au-naturel!) Jasmine is deliciously nourishing and is excellent for hot and dry skins. If the skin has a pitta redness to it then jasmine feels like a wonderful treat. Again, this is an absolute not an essential oil.

When their marriage was annulled after 14 years of being together, Josephine was distraught. She busied herself by building the gorgeous gardens at Malmaison where she was said to only wear the fragrance of violets. A much more innocent message given out to the world. When she died, Napoleon covered her grave with violet plants before going into exile and wore some of the flowers in his locket until he died. Violet leaf is benign in the extreme; it is nurturing to the most delicate skins. This is a very costly absolute, but it is so strong you will never, ever need more than one drop and it will last you for ever.

Frankincense you know. It is one of the hottest topics today, after the finding that the resin (<u>not the essential oil</u>) may be able to cure some types of cancer. The resin was used in the mummification of the pharaohs and even today there is no better preservative that I know of. Remember too, how dry and arid those Egyptian tombs would have been. Frankincense is for very dry skins; older skins if you like. It restores elasticity and so is wonderful for smoothing out wrinkles too.

Step away from the lavender if you have dry skin

So the first mistake people make with aromatherapy is they forget that essential oils do not have side effects, but instead they have many main effects. They lie in bath after bath of lavender to get them to sleep at night and then start to complain that their skin is drying out. The reason for this is lavender reduces the amount of sebum the skin makes.

This is great if you truly have a greasy teenager because we do want to calm the sebum and actually soothing the teenage angst is very helpful too. But if the skin is oily, rather than greasy teenager-y, then the orange tree has many gifts. Neroli if you can afford it, petitgrain, orange flower hydrolat...all fantastic astringents. We'll look more at astringents when we think about toners.

We have this same issue, really, with acne too. There can be a tendency to think of acne as teenage spots but it can last far longer through life, and actually it may not be that greasy at all. A mixture of tea tree to tackle any underlying infection and jasmine to nourish the skin and soothe the hot inflammation is a much better choice than lavender here.

A quick overview of the main skin care oils

Normal – Rose or geranium

Dry – rose

Mature - Frankincense

Oily – lavender - neroli

Combination – ylang ylang (it balances)

Sensitive - violet leaf or camomile

Acne – jasmine, tea tree.

Understanding Bases

This part is every bit as important as the essential oils, because if you get the base wrong then the skin will not get better.

Here is the rule:

If the skin is dry...it needs water.

If it looks dull and lifeless, it needs food.

Sounds obvious doesn't it? But the temptation will always to be to put oil onto dry skin...the sebum glands think there is enough and they stop producing.

Moisturisers

When it is hot, we water the plants. They need a drink. In fact, *we* have a glass of water, because we need a drink. We moisturise the skin, because it needs a drink. A moisturiser is a water based cream; it is light and fluffy. Do not confuse it with a nourishing cream.

Nourishing Creams

So where a moisturiser slakes the thirst of the epidermis, a nourishing cream feeds it. Consider it to be chicken soup for the face! When we make these we literally pack them with ingredients that will nourish the skin. They are thicker than moisturisers. A good skin care regime will include both of these, daily. I use my moisturiser twice a day and a nourishing cream at night, or as a base to make my cosmetics look several hundreds of pounds more expensive! It creates a glorious canvass to paint your war paint onto.

Large Scale Renovation!

I never quite "got" the point of rejuvenating creams until I had my blood clot and the medication I was on leeched every bit of vitality from my body and the my skin really suffered. They are like nourishing creams but are more like emergency first aid or to kick start a large scale renovation of seriously neglected complexion. Incidentally, if you have done that, don't panic or beat yourself up. I do it all the time. Life gets in the way. What I will tell you is this. The single biggest seller on Amazon about skin care is about how to treat yourself like a French woman, and how their attitudes about skin care are so different to ours. They look better because they *treat* themselves better. Skin care is a luxury that they believe their bodies deserve and they adore the process. I believe it...but can't do it!!! There is always a child who wants attention or some washing to do, or of course something I am bursting to type. Hence...I got good at putting my skin right...again!

I might be short, fat and the wrong side of forty, but my skin still looks beautiful thanks to some very specific oils.

Rejuvenating creams are too heavy to use for extended periods, but if you have been on medication for a long time, have been under stress or just want a mega boost before a hot date, a week of smearing your skin with this will make you über-confident about your ability to pull!

Creating a Bespoke Skin Care Formula

This is my attempt at not selling out entirely by giving you a book of recipes and so you never learn a thing. To do really excellent therapy it is impossible to use the same recipe over and over again. Everyone has skin issues arising from different things. For instance, mine is always weather beaten because of the wind and rain in the Shropshire hills. That means I am always peering in the mirror in expectation of broken capillaries too. My blood vessels are fragile after taking blood thinners for so long. There will be very few of you who have the same issues, and so emulating that is pointless so...

Tick all that apply

Fine lines		Frankincense
Wrinkles		Frankincense and galbanum
Blackheads		grapefruit
White heads		grapefruit
Open pores		myrtle
Redness		geranium
Hyper pigmentation		myrrh
Scarring		jasmine
Dark rings under the		Geranium

eyes		
Puffy eyes		Fennel, angelica
Loose and puffy skin		Frankincense and cypress

Adding just one single drop of the corresponding oil to your mix will tackle the specific problem for you.

A couple more tips:

Dark rings around the eyes, I am afraid your mum is right. Going to bed an hour earlier for a week is going to make a massive difference! For dark rings and puffy eyes though...a used camomile tea bag on your eyes for ten minutes works wonders...also if you have hay fever or sore eyes too.

Water: I am not going to labour the point, because we all know we should be drinking more water, but did you know when the body does not have enough reserves it starts to shut down supplies to various systems? The first system it deprives of water is the skin, prioritising supplies to the brain circulation and digestion. The single best thing you can do for the skin is to add some more water into you your diet each day.

Fruit Bowl Skin Care

As a pitta, the idea of a fast is like hell on a plate to me, but I have found moving over to juices-only for two or three days does miraculous things to my skin and hair. Potentially this has a lot to do with having more fluids, but also more vitamins too. The effects are dramatic and quick. Ladies and gentlemen...get yourselves a juicer! If you are wondering what to do with all the pulp left over...facemasks and fruit crumbles for when you go back onto solids again!

Here are some of my favourite fruits to either throw into a juicer or alternatively pack on my face...and make my kids squeal with laughter at me. (Rude, frankly!) These fruits are specifically chosen for being good for dry skins.

Apple

Apples are nourishing, hydrating and refreshing. They ooze vitamin C so are great for encouraging new cell growth and feeding the emerging cells beneath the surface. I grate them if I want to use them cold, but they are also wonderful stewed and then mixed with honey. Make sure you let them cool before you put them onto the skin though, because honey in particular can be spiteful when it is warm. Packed full of antioxidants this is a real anti-aging gift, especially if you will insist on killing the skin cells with cigarette smoke.

Banana

Now if you fancy a bit of Mickey Rourke action by the fridge, there simply cannot be a more 9 and half weeks ingredient than banana. Everything about it is rude. Mash it to soothe and smooth the skin. Perhaps this is something only the woman of a certain age would get! Given that it is absolutely oozing anti-aging vitamins, this one is a must.

Blueberries

Blueberries are great, but not too many too often, because they can be quite astringent. That aside, they smooth the skin and balance the sebum production. They increase circulation and reduce broken capillaries and spider veins.

Dragon fruit

The bright pink monsters in the fruit aisle are like a Niagara Falls of hydration. Consisting of around 80% water they flood the skin like no other fruit can. They are very soothing too, so of you happen to have been scorched by dragon's breath, or if you have become sunburnt or have eczema, this is a great big aaaah moment of relief!

Lychees

Once in a while, five minutes soaking up a bit of lychee can be very beneficial. They are very astringent so they great cleansers slicing through grease and grime. The skin is also toned and tightened by their juices.

Mango

Mango is the menopausal goddess's best friend. Aging loosens the elasticity in the skin, which causes wrinkles. Mango picks up the slack making the skin far more taut and smooth.

Orange

Oranges are full of collagen so are wonderful for mature skins. Use them dried to make fabulous scrubs! Fresh, they a bit too acidic to put on the skin, I feel.

Papaya

There is an enzyme in papaya which strips away dead cells and clears away impurities. It is a must have for scrubs and masques.

Pineapple

This is a really important fruit to fight the onset of aging. Its component alpha-hydroxl acid tightens wrinkles and helps to alleviate warts and moles. The acids though are very acidic so

only leave on for about 3 minutes. By five minutes you should expect a chemical burn so bad that it can make the skin bleed.

Pears

My very favourite fruit to eat and to use on my skin. Pears nourishing to your skin and balance excess sebum production too. An excellent choice if you have combination skin. They make lovely masques, but their granular texture also works well in facial scrubs too.

Peach

Peaches are a dry skin's very best friend. In particular, use the juice for a nourishment treatment. Add a tea spoon to a masque for instance...and try not to lick it all off!

Pomegranate

A bit of pomegranate in a scrub is fabulous. The juice is astringent, cleansing and tightening. Massaging the seeds against the skin sloughs off old dead skins, revealing younger fresher cells beneath. Facial circulation loves it!

Raspberry

Raspberries are an extra special gift. My dad used to grow them in the allotment when I was a child. It always grieves me to have to pay for them now! It is worth it though, because they charm the circulation and bring colour and glow to dull and lifeless skins.

Strawberry

Strawberries hydrate the skin with bucketfuls of vitamin C. It is like turning the taps on your skin's moisture switch.

If you are making a fruit masque you will need a powdered stabiliser. You can use the clays recommended in the masques section, but I find the following powders to be just as good for dry skin

- Oatmeal
- Wheatgerm
- Gram Flour (made of chick peas)
- Dried Milk

Also natural yoghurt!

I always slip in a tea spoon of honey and also a tea spoon of sesame oil into warm masques to give them real life and vitality.

Warm or Cold?

It doesn't really matter which. Go with the flow and what you have in the house or you see festering in the reduced aisle of the supermarket really! Warm masques will open the pores and let the goodness in and would delight vata and kapha constitutions. A cold masque will cease pores closed and of course that traps in the moisture and tones the skin. Both are beneficial. Hence when I am being a good girl, I do one of each!

I won't give you too many recipes here, because really it is chuck it all in the bowl and see what comes out!

A couple of examples though...

Warm Natural Face Pack

1 tbs wheatgerm

1 tbs dried milk powder

½ mashed banana

6 strawberries

1 stewed pear

Directions:

Chop the pear up into small pieces and then stew slowly in a 3 fl oz of water.

Cook tall softened then removed with a slotted spoon

Add the mashed banana and smashed strawberries

Stir in honey and sesame oil

Then add enough dry ingredients to bring together into a manageable paste.

Smear on and leave on the skin for about 8 minutes

Tissue off and then rinse with warm water. Tone and cleanse the pores with rosewater.

Cold Natural face pack

½ Mashed Mango

¼ Mashed dragon fruit

¼ Mashed papaya

1 tbs milk powder

Throw it all in the liquidiser and blitz or grate together.

Use on the skin for about 8 minutes.

Tissue off and close pores with a toner to seal in all of that lovely hydration

Skin Care Products

In every recipes I will delineate how many drops of essential oils thus:

X 1 = 1 drop

X 2 = 2 drops

X 3 = 3 drops

You can work the rest out!

Cleansers

I have to say, I have never been able to find a recipe for a cleanser base that did not make my skin drier, because it contained soap. Therefore then, I always go to the supermarket and buy the cheapest one I can find and then adulterate it to make it better.

The advantage to do this is that it comes in a readymade bottle. The downside is that essential oils will, over time, eat through the bottle so I would always recommend finding a beautiful glass bottle and decanting it.

Rehydration for very thirsty skin
50 ml blank cleanser

Geranium x 1

Frankincense x 1

Vetiver x 1

City Slickers Cleanser

If you live in the city and are dodging the traffic then all manner of air borne pollutants settle on the skin. These free radicals are very harmful to skin cells causing it to oxidise. This leads to premature aging. One of the first signs you will see is dryness and then I am afraid wrinkles will follow.

Let's remove them now...

50ml (2 fl oz) blank cleanser

3 x carrot seed oil

1 x cypress

1 x parsley seed

Commercial Cream

If you work in an office, then you are surrounded by absolutely everything bad for your skin. Computers emit positive ions, fluorescent bulbs glare and the air con saps every bit of moisture from your skin. Potentially too, your perfectly set make up hides a multitude of sins because your poor skin gets no time to breathe. Cleansing all this environmental pollution quickly yields results.

50ml (2 fl oz) blank cleanser

3 x cypress

1 x patchouli

1 neroli

Toners

The purpose of the toning fluid is to close the pores and to tighten the skin. They are beautifully refreshing and I find they are lovely for getting rid of the last of the cleanser or masque.

When I do a facial, I will use a toner after each different product. It is a beautifully sensuous aspect because things like facial massage stimulate the circulation and make the complexion very warm. Being drenched in a cool, fragrant wash is one of my very favourite things.

You will recall that essential oils and water don't mix and this will cause you some issues making toner. You could add a teaspoon of vodka to the blend but it will probably make your skin drier.

There is a small amount of alcohol in witch hazel blends that is functional here and again I love the coolness it provides. Your pharmacist is likely to have some behind the counter he can sell you. I tend not to add any essential oils to my toners these days and simply use pure unadulterated rosewater. Why pollute perfection in my opinion!

Floral waters, or hydrolats are bi-products of the extraction of essential oils. As steam is passed through the plant matter it collects the oil, then it is cooled and condensed. The oil floats on top of the water and is separated off for us to buy. The water though, contains tiny particulates of the oil and is a gentler form of the oil. Hydrolats make the perfect toners in my opinion.

But if you do want to play with your oils...here are a few ideas for you.

City Toner
This is designed to go along with the cleansers for the environmental pollutants

50ml (2 fl oz) orange flower water (also known as neroli hydrolat)

25ml (1tsp) witch hazel

Petitgrain x 1

Carrot x 1

Cypress x 1

Toner for mature skins
50 ml frankincense hydrolat

25 ml witch hazel

1 x frankincense

1 x galbanum

1 x myrrh

Toner for hot, sore skins
25ml (1tsp) rose water

25 ml yarrow hydrolat

25 ml with hazel

1 x violet leaf absolute

1 x camomile roman

Egyptian Luxury
In my book Rose – A Goddess Medicine, I describe how
Cleopatra sailed down the river to meet Mark Anthony, the
sails of her ship doused with precious oils. I make this recipe

to try to emulate the scent I suspected would have drifted on the winds that day. No wonder he was smitten!

25 ml Rosewater

25 ml orange flower water

1/3 tsp vodka

Myrrh x 1

Galbanum x 1

Rose x 1

Because the myrrh and galbanum are thick, base note fixatives, you are going to need to dissolve them first. I use an egg cup, and drop the oils into the vodka, give it a quick squizz with the wrong end of a tea spoon then pour it into the hydrolats.

Each different season offers up their own challenges. As I write this I am stranded in the shed because of monsoon-like conditions which certainly should not belong to a British August. Yesterday though, was hot and dry and my skin was parched by the end of the day. In winter, the wind is harsh and bitter here and that ravages my already red complexion making it hot and sore. So let's think about some ways of counteracting those....

Summertime salve

50 ml Palmarosa hydrolat

10 ml Witch hazel

Geranium x 1

Camomile x 1

Patchouli x 1

Winter Ravaged Skin

Deliciously spicy and warming for those days when you would rather be sitting by the fire (A whole new dimension to drying out your skin!!!)

25 ml Sandalwood hydrolat

15 ml Camomile Roman hydrolat

10 ml witch hazel

Cardamom x 1

Yarrow x 1

Palmarosa x 1

Facial Scrubs

The top layer of your skin is comprised of dead skin cells. By sloughing the top layer, we reveal younger fresher cells. Exfoliation also helps to alleviate issues such as blocked pores and black heads too. Most importantly, as well as a fresher more translucent complexion your skin feels smooth and soft.

Essentially these are abrasive and scratch away the dead skin. Unlike body scrubs that are made of salts and hard sugars, I find facial scrubs made of soft sugars and cereals work best. Molasses or Demerara are gorgeous - the softer the better.) Don't worry about scrubbing too hard either. Gentle circles work well because we will continue the exfoliation with the facial massage oils later.

Here, it would be criminal to use absolutes and our top end essential oils because they are but moments on the skin, so, I like to get creative with bits and pieces I have made from the garden.

Hazelnut is always my preferred carrier oil because it is by far the best exfoliator. If you are allergic to nuts though, I would opt for rosehip or evening primrose. You can of course use olive or sunflower if that's all you have!

Rose Petal Renaissance
25g wheatgerm

1 tsp of soft brown sugar

10g dried rose petals

1 tsp hazelnut oil

Camomile Calmer

25g oatmeal

1 tsp soft brown sugar

10 g camomile flowers

1 tsp hazelnut oil

Blackhead Buster

25g oatmeal

1 tsp soft brown sugar

10 g dried orange and grapefruit peels grated or chopped into tiny pieces

1 tsp hazelnut oil

Scrub for Sensitive Skin

15g oatmeal

10g dried milk powder

1 tsp soft brown sugar

10 g dried lavender and camomile flowers

1 tsp hazelnut oil

Smoker's Skins

This is thicker, richer and more abrasive to really work the worn out skin.

25g wheat germ

1 tsp of soft brown sugar

10g mix of dried rose petals, lavender and camomile

1 tsp hazelnut oil

½ tsp borage oil

Facial Massage Oil

Here is where the magic lives because the smallest gentles movements are going to relax all that tension in your face as well as smoothing away dead cells and invigorating circulation. In Ayurveda, this part is called *oleation*...meaning we have oiled the skin. Oleation followed by steam is a fundamental Ayurvedic principle in the treatment of dry skin. We oil it then we open the pores to let the oil penetrate deeply into the tissues.

One of the first things I teach students about massage is to listen to their fingers. You will find out everything you need to know about the problems in the face by what you feel under your finger tips. Where is it rough? Where are you holding tension? Are there bumps threatening to turn into blemishes?

Be in tune with your skin.

You are going to do the same massage twice in two different ways. Only use your fingertips and first, you want to work the muscles so you are using a slightly harder pressure and this means your fingers hardly slide on the skins surface at all. Muscle tissues are made up of many fibres and on the face they all cross over each other to make all your facial expression work. Lifting and separating the fibres is very relaxing. Simply releasing stress from your face can take ten years off you.

The second massage is all very light touch and this time we are looking to slide across the skin and let the oil take away the dead cells.

Facial massage is covered in depth in my free book *The Complete Guide...* but very basically you are making tiny circles on the flesh with your fingertips. Start at the middle of forehead, right at the hairline and work outwards. Make line after line of tiny circles, coming down the forehead, then onto the cheeks and chin. Really work the oil into grimy places like the chin and the nose and you will find that you can feel the cells become gritty under your fingers as they come away. It is worth bringing the massage down onto the neck and shoulders. Squeeze away the tension and really feel yourself relax.

Again here, I always use hazelnut oil to exfoliate and sesame to nourish and warm vata. Wheatgerm oil is not only bursting with vitamin E to nourish the skin but it also magically boosts the effects of the other oils. Which other carrier oils you add to that is entirely up to you

Deep Relaxation

Rose x 1

Sandalwood x 1

Yarrow x 1

Dehydrated Skin

Rose x 1

Geranium x 1

Cedarwood x 1

Mature Skin

Frankincense x 1

Galbanum x 1

Vetiver x 1

Combination Skin

Ylang ylang x 1

Geranium x 1

Cypress x 1

Dry Puffy Face

Angelica x 1

Cypress x 1

Geranium x 1

After one of hell of a week at the office
Carrot x 1

Cypress x 1

Geranium x 1

Frankincense x 1

Steam Cleanse

OOOO, my absolute favourite. You can spend what you like on a cleanser but it will never get the skin as clean as one of these. I recommend doing them weekly, no more than that though. The idea is to use the warmth to open the pores and then the sweat brings the dirt locked under the skin out. If you doubt that there is any take a look at your skin before and after, it literally changes colour as the debris pours out.

These are the perfect pick me up if you have a cold too, because not only do you feel rubbish, but you look bad too. A few minutes over the steam clears your nose and improves the skin!!!

Winners all round.

These are so simple, and sometimes I just use herbs that I haven't quite used up from making dinner as well as, or instead of, oils. Chuck them in, it all adds to the mix! What I will say is herbs and flowers work better than spices I find, which are a bit too harsh somehow.

Your receptacle doesn't need to be large. I use a pudding basin. Fill it with boiling water then add your oils. You will need to make a tent over your head to trap the steam in. Keep your face about 8 ins away from the water. The last thing you want to do is scald yourself.

I will say, this treatment can make you feel dizzy, so if you start to feel light headed...stop. Try again in a few minutes if you want to.

A treatment usually lasts about 5 – 7 minutes.

Taking a steam, can be a bit oppressive for some people, and actually does not work very well in a clinical setting. Here then, we replace with a warm compress. Take a cloth, a tea towel works well, and cut out holes for the eyes nose and mouth. Soak in the prepared oiled water, and then ring out. Making sure it is not too hot for the skin; lay it onto the face to open the pores, for about 5 minutes.

When you have finished, wash your towel out immediately. Dry, and put away to use next time.

Incidentally, don't forget to consider the emotional effects of each blend of oils. They are not only going to clean your skin but they will affect your mood too.

Geranium steam cleanse
Mellowwww....

Geranium x 1

Ylang ylang x 1

Carrot x 1

Neroli Steam Cleanse
Happy, *happy,* **happy**...Goodbye worries! Come on world...bring it on!!!!

Neroli x 1

Basil x 1

Litsea Cubeba (May Chang) x 1

Sensuous Rose

Feed your skin and give your self esteem a mega boost with this blend

Rose otto x 1

Ylang Ylang x 1

Vetiver x 1

Summer Salad

Refreshing and Deeply Cleansing

Carrot seed x1

Parsley seed x 1

Thyme x 1

Relax and soothe

Drift away in a summer's garden

Lavender x 1

Camomile x 1

Geranium x 1

Moisturisers

Before we start: a quick note on glycerine. It is an animal derived product but if you ask the pharmacist he should be able to supply you with vegetable glycerine if you prefer. It is actually a substance for making sweets so you can usually get it on the cake/candy making aisle of the supermarket.

Its function in the skin treatment is to draw moisture up to the surface of the skin from deeper tissues. This is very useful in the UK and one day I hope that my face will benefit from the fluid being drawn off my hips but...if you like somewhere very hot, it might not be the best plan to include it. After all your internal organs are going to need all the hydration they can get.

Glycerine makes up just 2% of the finished formula so if you decide to omit it, simply add 1% to your water calculation and 1%to your carrier oil. Do not up your essential oil quota it will be too harsh.

I use aqueous cream as the beginning of my cream. I checked: you can buy this off Amazon in the States. I get mine from the local chemist and from Aldi. Keep your eyes peeled for deals.

Lastly a quick comment about essential oils that really applies right through the book, but it is particularly pertinent here.

Your maximum dilution for oils is 3%. Many of these recipes don't even go that high, because you simply don't need to.

Moisturiser recipe

For ease, we'll use a whole 500g tub. That will make about 20 x 50ml (2 fl oz) jars. That should give you a good start on the Christmas presents! Incidentally, don't feel you have to add the essential oils in at this point. You can always make a "blank" mix and then add different oils to each pot.

If you want to make a single pot though, just do half aqueous and half water then add one drop of each oil you want. ½ tsp of glycerine should be ample.

500ml aqueous cream

450 ml water

30 ml essential oils

20ml glycerine

Use a hand whisk to bind together

Simple as! But the real skill comes from how you adapt that and make it your own.

For instance....water? We could change that into rose water, or peony tea! Think your recipe through before you start. The essential oils will make it lovely but carrier oils and floral waters you add make it exceptional! Bear in mind too...if you make a cup of strong Yorkshire Tea...you will have a brown cream which is not very pleasant! Jasmine tea is fabulous as is chrysanthemum or green tea. Likewise you can make infusions from any plants in the garden. That ridiculous sticky grass, cleavers? Wondrous for the skin. Leave it to steep in hot water for 2 hours and add the water. Rose flowers, violets or yarrow flowers for example all make beautiful infusions that you can add instead of just water.

A word to the wise...let the tea cool before you add it!

The same applies for carrier oils, of course. Get out into the garden and fill your sunflower oil with calendula flowers, rose petals or jasmine blooms and leave them to steep for a month! These are a fraction of the price of shop bought carriers and you have the added pleasure of knowing you have created something magical yourself.

Exquisite rose moisturiser for normal and combination skins
100g (4oz) aqueous cream

70 ml (2 ½ fl oz) Rosehip tea (steeped for 3 mins, then left to cool with tea bags removed)

25 ml (1 fl oz) rose hydrolat

1ml rosehip carrier oil

2ml (1/2 tsp) glycerine

5ml (1tsp) (1 tsp) wheatgerm oil

Rose absolute x 1

Ylang ylang x 2

Geranium x 1

Mix together gently, until well combined. Divide between 4 sterilised jars and cap immediately.

Hot Sore Skin
100g (4oz) aqueous cream

70 ml (2 ½ fl oz) Camomile tea (steeped for 3 mins, then left to cool with tea bags removed)

25 ml (1 fl oz) rose hydrolat

1ml calendula carrier oil

2ml (1/2 tsp) glycerine

5ml (1tsp) (1 tsp) wheatgerm oil

Patchouli x 1

Camomile x 2

Sandalwood x 2

10ml (2tsp) calendula oil

5ml (1tsp) wheatgerm oil

Mix together gently, until well combined. Divide between 4 sterilised jars and cap immediately.

Frankincense Froth

This is a beautiful blend for more mature skins, to restore elasticity and to bring a bloom back to the skin.

100g (4oz) aqueous cream

70 ml (2 ½ fl oz) Raspberry Leaf tea (steeped for 3 mins, then left to cool with tea bags removed)

25 ml (1 fl oz) Frankincense hydrolat

1ml Evening Primrose carrier oil

2ml (1/2 tsp) glycerine

5ml (1tsp) (1 tsp) wheatgerm oil

Frankincense x 1

Camomile x 2

Myrrh x 2

Mix together gently, until well combined. Divide between 4 sterilised jars and cap immediately.

Weather Beaten Skin

100g (4oz) aqueous cream

70 ml (2 ½ fl oz) Jasmine tea (steeped for 3 mins, then left to cool with tea bags removed)

25 ml (1 fl oz) jasmine hydrolat

5 ml (1tsp) evening primrose carrier oil

5 ml (1 tsp) almond carrier oil

2ml (1/2 tsp) glycerine

5ml (1tsp) (1 tsp) wheatgerm oil

Cardamom x 2

Patchouli x 2

Rose absolute x 1

Mix together gently, until well combined. Divide between 4 sterilised jars and cap immediately.

Masculine Moisturiser

This blend pulls together the gifts of the rose to feed and nourish the skin but over lays their fragrance with deeply sensuous and masculine fragrances. Deliciously earthy food for the skin.

100g (4oz) aqueous cream

70 ml (2 ½ fl oz) Rosehip Tea (steeped for 3 mins, then left to cool with tea bags removed)

25 ml (1 fl oz) jasmine hydrolat

5 ml (1 tsp) Sesame carrier oil

5 ml (1 tsp) Rosehip carrier oil

2ml (1/2 tsp) glycerine

5ml (1tsp) (1 tsp) wheatgerm oil

Cardamom x 2

Patchouli x 2

Sandalwood x 1

Nourishing Creams

Now I am going to be very English here and make the first set of measurements in metric. It is easier to calculate percentages, so I'll show you how to calculate that way first and then we can move over to imperial.

Primary school science taught us that oil and water don't mix. It is true. You can make them blend though, if you add an emulsifier. There are many of these on the market, but the simplest and easiest to use is labelled "Emulsifying wax". Others are also labelled *cetearyl alcohol* and *polysorbate 60.*

From now on I shall call it E/W.

How much E/W you add to a cream will determine its consistency.

Add 2-5% for a lotion

Add 5-7% for creams

Add 10-15% for body butters.

I use a ratio of:

55% water base

33% oil

2% glycerine

7% E/W

3% Essential oils (E/O)

Recipe for a Nourishing Cream

To make a litre of face cream (which is obviously 20 x 50ml (2 fl oz) pots)

550 ml (19 fl oz) water

330 ml (12 fl oz) oil

20 ml (1 tbs) glycerine

70 g (2 ½ oz) Emulsifying wax

30 ml (1 fl oz) essential oils (approx 600 drops total is probably easier)

Take your E/W and place into a bain marie. Allow it to warm and melt in its own time over a medium heat.

Boil the kettle and measure out your boiling water.

Pour the meted E/W and water into a food processor, add the carrier oil and mix.

Watch your mixture. You want it well mixed, but not full of air otherwise it will sink when it cools. I find it easiest to pulse the blender.

If you are adding E/Os now, drop them in and give one more quick blitz to ensure they are blended.

Use a jug to pour into sterilised jars

Leave to cool thoroughly before you put the tops on. If you rush, I can absolutely guarantee you it will go mouldy on the top!

Preservatives

There are preservatives that you can add to your creams such as Germaben II (which is some kind of paraben derivative), but I prefer to keep things au-natural, and for the most part essential oils will act as preservatives, especially if you have antifungal oils like tea tree in the blend of course.

Keeping your pots of cream small will help, because obviously you will use them up more quickly. If you do have spares you can always pop them in the fridge as long as you label them clearly. I have a very steamy warm bathroom and a cream doesn't last more than a few weeks in there. Storing somewhere cool is better.

It is most definitely easier if you make a larger batch than a smaller one. Even more so, you can make lots of "blank" creams (with no essential oils in them) and then make each one separately.

This also works very well if you want to do Christmas gifts because you can get 20 done in one afternoon!!!

Simply add into your 50 ml pot. If you do decide to add all your essential oils into a master mix, you will need to multiply your oils quantities by 20.

Midnight Garden

Geranium x 1

Jasmine x 1

Vetiver x 1

Spirit of Oberon

Strong, sexy and very enigmatic. This blend is for the male who knows how important looking good can be.

Sandalwood x 1

Cedarwood x 1

Patchouli x 1

Camomile x 1

Sensitive Salve

Camomile x 1

Violet Leaf x 1

Melissa x 1

Over Fifties Face Feast!

Rose x 1

Frankincense x 1

Sandalwood x 1

Angelica x 1

Extra Special Skin Delight
Rose x 2

Cypress x 1

Patchouli x 1

Jasmine x 2

Masques

Now, you can spend a pretty penny on face masque bases...and sometimes I do. But I have to admit the best ones I find are either made from bits and pieces that I haven't managed to use up from the fruit bowl or from clays.

I like clays a lot!!! I also like seaweeds which are also very good at pulling out impurities. What I don't like is the mess they make. You have been warned!!! They get everywhere. They stain towels, so use old ones and don't even think about leaving the bathroom without cleaning the sink because it is harder to get off the basin than yesterday's porridge!!!

But...

Who doesn't love mud pies.....?

For dry skin use RED CLAY to nourish and KAOLIN to cleanse and draw impurities.

Somehow clay feels absolutely aligned to aromatherapy, coming from the ground. Red clay is volcanic soil. It is packed with vital minerals and nutrients and really feeds the skin. It will also draw out toxins that are deep below the surface. To use it in its simplest form you simply mix with water (see I told you it was mud pies!) but we can improve on that so much if we add oils.

If you want to give this as a gift, pack it in two parts; the clay in a little packet and then your blended oil. You use about a dessert spoon full of clay for a treatment with enough oil to blend it into a paste.

The following recipes are for the oils to stir into the red clay.

Soothing Masque
Gentle enough for conditions such as eczema or psoriasis or even very sensitive skins.

1 tsp sea buckthorn C/O

1 tsp evening primrose C/O

Rose x 1

Violet leaf x 1

Camomile Matricaria x 1

Weekly Revive
1 tsp rosehip C/O

1 tsp wheatgerm C/O

Geranium x 1

Patchouli

Sandalwood

After Illness and Long Term Stress
1 tsp borage C/O

Holy Basil x 1

Vetiver x 1

Helichrysm x 1

Allergic Skin
1 tsp Calendula C/O

Melissa x 1

Violet leaf x 1

Camomile Roman x 1

Revitalisation Treatments
Sometimes we need something extra. Perhaps after we have been poorly, or after a week of solid climbing the hill in the

snow, for instance! You know those days when you look in the mirror and you groan!!! These are emergency first aid creams for days when you look seriously scary!!!

By now you should be getting the hang of how we make the changes. We up the emulsifier first so the nourishing cream becomes a thicker base, and I also replace some of the oil with a butter...shea butter, cocoa butter take your pick. **Coconut oil** makes it **<u>lovely and light</u>** and **shea butter** is **thick and nurturing**. My local organic shop sells lots of these butters and if you can get your hands on them you can really make some fab changes. Brazil nut butter is my favourite.

Another more costly way of making these is to source some floral waxes. I talk about these extensively in my book, *Rose Goddess Medicine*. They are a bi-product of the process of making absolutes. They are not cheap but they make sublime creams. You are usually looking about £10/$15 for 2oz depending on what plant you source from. I have to say they do not carry much scent, so they won't fragrance your cream per se, but they will improve the texture and bring the properties of the plants. The maximum quantity you will want to add is 10% of your mix. Warm them slowly and add them into the oil part of the mix.

50% water base

25% oil

8% butter / wax

2% glycerine

12% E/W

3% essential oils

Some blends then...

I'll make these as 100g (4oz blends)

Master Protector

A gem for slathering all over your face before you encounter the elements each day. Because the wax content is higher it will sit on your skin and form a protective barrier against the wind and rain.

50ml (2 fl oz) (2 fl oz) rosewater

10ml (2tsp) rosehip c/o

10ml (2tsp) jojoba c/o

5ml (1tsp) wheatgerm oil

1 tsp shea butter

½ tsp rose wax

12ml (1 fl oz) E/W

2ml (1/2) tsp glycerine

Patchouli x 5

Geranium x 5

Sandalwood x 3

Cardamom x 3

Camomile roman x 5

Instructions

Take your E/W and place into a bain marie. Allow it to warm and melt in its own time over a medium heat.

Boil the kettle and measure out your boiling water.

Melt the butter and wax together VERY slowly ensuring that they don't start to fry, as they start to soften add the carrier oil to warm and combine.

Pour the meted E/W and water into a food processor, add the oil/butter mix, then the glycerine and blend together.

Watch your mixture. You want it well mixed, but not full of air otherwise it will sink when it cools. I find it easiest to pulse the blender.

If you are adding E/Os now, drop them in and give one more quick blitz to ensure they are blended.

Use a jug to pour into sterilised jars

Leave to cool thoroughly before you put the tops on. If you rush, I can absolutely guarantee you it will go mouldy on the top!

Poorly Bird Salve!

For days when your nose looks like someone has scraped it raw and you wonder if you will ever look pretty again!

50ml (2 fl oz) camomile hydrolat

10ml (2tsp) evening primrose c/o

5ml (1tsp) olive c/o

5ml (1tsp) rosehip c/o

5ml (1tsp) wheatgerm oil

1 tsp shea butter

½ tsp jasmine wax

12ml (1 fl oz) E/W

2ml (1/2) tsp glycerine Lavender x 2

Holy basil x 2

Rose x 2

Geranium x 6

Sandalwood x 6

Vetiver x 1

Click for Instructions

Packaging

I won't patronise you by telling you how to design packaging. I actually think part of the charm is that your personality really shines through by the colours you add to the labels and the overall image you portray. That part, I can't teach you. This is where your natural flare should burst from your pot.

All I will say is your oils will stay active for longer in dark glass. Brown can be made beautiful and it is possible to get pinks, blues, reds and green glasses if you look hard enough.

Have a look at websites who sell essential oils, they usually have jars too. I have found lovely ones on Ebay and Amazon and don't discount vintage shops either. There is no rule that says everything has to match.

It is possible to get aluminium, lined, bottles which I adore and they look super modern and sassy. Plastic ones, guys and gals, just won't do. They just collapse after a couple of days with oils in them.

I thought you might enjoy this little tool that makes professional looking labelling a cinch.

http://www.jamlabelizer.com/

Some of the designs are free, some you have to pay $8 membership for. It is very cute and easy to use. If you go to the local stationary shop and ask the man for a single A4 label, you can print onto it and cut out your design.

I'll state the obvious here, because it usually takes me three weeks for the penny to drop on these sorts of things...

Temptation might creep in for you to say you want to label your cream "Grandma's Skin Cream" and "Auntie Jean's Face Cream" when you see what the tool can do. It is, however a much better plan to call it "The Secret Healer's Cream" or whatever name you choose, because you will have a whole sheet all the same and you will be paying for stacks of wastage if you are not careful.

Labelling

This is another book in its own right that someone *else* can write! But...

If you are making creams for yourself or as gifts then, knock yourself out, call them anything you like. If you intend to sell them, however, you need to be careful about your labelling. Now these are not so contentious because, you can make cosmetic claims and say it is for dry skin, but if you veer over to "Eczema" then you are breaking the law. You cannot say that unless your product has been medically licensed, or you have had a one to one consultation with your client (and you are a qualified therapist). You also need to list all ingredients in the tub (or on an attached leaflet enclosed in the packaging).

Safest then is to make up silly names for them like..

Spirit of Oberon! Dry Skin Delight etc etc

Conclusion...

Actually, this is but the start, because now I have to write all the other skin types, don't I?

I nearly opened the book with a quote by Anne Roife who said: *A woman whose smile is open and whose expression is glad has a kind of beauty no matter what she wears.* I think this is absolutely true because true happiness is the very healthiest face you can wear. There is no greater tool to help you with this than aromatherapy. Make sure you are getting your daily dose of rose coloured glasses and a good dose of Sweet Basil enthusiasm every day. Please make the very best use of my book The Essential Oils of The Mind Body Spirit. It will give you look in the mirror in a whole different way. If you look terrible, I promise you your body is warning you about something...

You absolutely must take heed.

As ever, thanks so much for buying and reading and I would love it if you would please leave me a review. Just before I go, I want to give my little sister Angela, to whom this book is dedicated) a wave. Actually she is my step sister, so this part of life is a fairly new discovery to her and she has started to experiment making her own little pots of cream. In her day job she is a fabulous midwife and by evenings and weekends she and her husband are working towards having a self-sufficient life away from the rat race. She has a little candle and crafts website: http://www.pilipala.biz/has bought a piece of woodland and breeds the most incredible Ayam Cemani chickens. So Ang, this book is for you, to say I love you, and thank you for your never ending support. I am so proud you are following in the family tradition and I hope one day to buy a pot of cream off you, in a shop nestled in woodland surrounded by wonderful black chucks!!!! Please know that every one of your dreams is my dream for you too.

Over the next few weeks, please look out for my other books in The Secret Healer Beauty Tips Series for:

- Oily Skin
- Sensitive Skin and Rosacea
- Acne

As well as a manual of tips about how to use your essential oils to make exquisite and cost effective handmade gifts.

But for now, happy skin care and remember

Review and Buy! Bye!

Liz x

About the Author

Elizabeth Ashley qualified as an aromatherapist in 1993, and then passed her Advanced Aromatherapy Diploma in 1994. She has been practicing aromatherapy for almost 22 years.

In 1999, she fell into a whole new career in the aggressive commercial sector of recruitment consultancy. There she discovered her father's second hand car salesman genes had passed along and found she had quite a gift of the gab! More than that, she discovered she could sell...and then some.

In 2008, Elizabeth fell ill during pregnancy with a blood clot in her lungs. The pulmonary embolism prevented her from working and she started to write. Very quickly she gained her first contract as a ghost writer...a recipe book for cheese cakes!

In 2010 she was published professionally for her work on Galbanum oil in the Aromatherapy Thymes, journal of the International Federation of Aromatherapists, and on Tuberose oil by the New Zealand Register of Holistic Therapist.

In 2011 she was seconded on a consultative basis to Walsall Independent Treatment Centre, designed to be a rainbow bridge between traditional and complementary medicines. There she became aware of the rumblings of change in healthcare. Her book *Sales Strategies for Gentle Souls* explains the connotations of this.

Many of her books are aimed at helping qualified aromatherapists to expand their healing repertoire and build their businesses. She also writes for people who have an interest in essential oils and want to learn how to heal. Her in depth essential oil profiles chart the healing properties of plants from the most arcane depths of historic folklore up to the scientific lab trials of today.

In 2014 she ranks in the top 50 contract writers on the freelancer marketplace Elance.com. She is the ghost writer of seven number one Amazon best sellers in the natural healing category. She lives in Shropshire with her husband and youngest son, kept company by their cat, the budgie and many shoals of tropical fish! Her elder son and daughter attend University and make her prouder than anything ever could.

Elizabeth Ashley is possibly one of the most published aromatherapy writers you have never heard of! By 2015, all of that will have changed. Elizabeth Ashley is *The Secret Healer*.

The Secret Healer Oils Profiles:

Some of the oils we have covered in this book will be familiar, but possibly not all. You may find some of the oils profiles deepen your knowledge and fascination for the art of aromatherapy.

Vetiver: the Oil of Tranquillity

Monarda: A Native American Medicine

Holy Basil: An Ayurvedic Medicine

Rose: Goddess Medicine; A Timeless Elixir

Sweet Basil – The Oil of Empowerment

The Secret Healing Manuals:

Book 1 - The Complete Guide to

Clinical Aromatherapy & Essential Oils for the Physical Body

Download for FREE

Book 2 Essential Oils for Mind Body Spirit

The Holistic Medicine of Clinical Aromatherapy

Book 3 The Essential Oil Liver Cleanse

The Professional Aromatherapist's Liver Detox

Book 4 The Professional Stress Solution

Essential Oils and Holistic Health Stress Management Techniques for The Professional Aromatherapist

Book 5 The Aromatherapy Eczema Treatment

Healing Eczema, Itchy Skin Rashes and Atopic Dermatitis with Essential Oils and Holistic Medicine

Book 6 The Aromatherapy Bronchitis Treatment

Support the Respiratory System with Essential Oils and Holistic Medicine for COPD, Emphysema, Acute and Chronic Bronchitis Symptoms

Sales Strategies for Gentle Souls

Targeted Sales Training for Professional Aromatherapists

www.thesecrethealer.co.uk

www.buildyourownreality.com

Disclaimer

by SEQ Legal

(1)   Introduction

This disclaimer governs the use of this book. [By using this book, you accept this disclaimer in full. / We will ask you to agree to this disclaimer before you can access the book.]

(2)   Credit

This disclaimer was created using an SEQ Legal template.

(3)   No advice

The book contains information about aromatherapy and the use of essential oils.The information is not advice, and should not be treated as such.

[You must not rely on the information in the book as an alternative to qualified medical advice from a health professional. advice from an appropriately qualified professional. If you have any specific questions about any medical matter you should consult an appropriately qualified professional.]

[If you think you may be suffering from any medical condition you should seek immediate medical attention. You should never delay seeking medical advice, disregard medical advice, or discontinue medical treatment because of information in the book.]

(4)   No representations or warranties

To the maximum extent permitted by applicable law and subject to section 6 below, we exclude all representations, warranties, undertakings and guarantees relating to the book.

Without prejudice to the generality of the foregoing paragraph, we do not represent, warrant, undertake or guarantee:

that the information in the book is correct, accurate, complete or non-misleading;

that the use of the guidance in the book will lead to any particular outcome or result; or in particular, that by using the guidance in the book you will heal disease or work in any way as a cure for illness.

(5)   Limitations and exclusions of liability

The limitations and exclusions of liability set out in this section and elsewhere in this disclaimer: are subject to section 6 below; and govern all liabilities arising under the disclaimer or in relation to the book, including liabilities arising in contract, in tort (including negligence) and for breach of statutory duty.

We will not be liable to you in respect of any losses arising out of any event or events beyond our reasonable control.

We will not be liable to you in respect of any business losses, including without limitation loss of or damage to profits, income, revenue, use, production, anticipated savings, business, contracts, commercial opportunities or goodwill.

We will not be liable to you in respect of any loss or corruption of any data, database or software.

We will not be liable to you in respect of any special, indirect or consequential loss or damage.

(6)   Exceptions

Nothing in this disclaimer shall: limit or exclude our liability for death or personal injury resulting from negligence; limit or exclude our liability for fraud or fraudulent misrepresentation; limit any of our liabilities in any way that is not permitted under applicable law; or exclude any of our liabilities that may not be excluded under applicable law.

(7)   Severability

If a section of this disclaimer is determined by any court or other competent authority to be unlawful and/or unenforceable, the other sections of this disclaimer continue in effect.

If any unlawful and/or unenforceable section would be lawful or enforceable if part of it were deleted, that part will be deemed to be deleted, and the rest of the section will continue in effect.

(8)   Law and jurisdiction

This disclaimer will be governed by and construed in accordance with English law, and any disputes relating to this disclaimer will be subject to the exclusive jurisdiction of the courts of England and Wales.

(9)   Our details

In this disclaimer, "we" means (and "us" and "our" refer to) [*Build Your Own Reality)*] of [*Sy8 1LQ*].

Made in the USA
Columbia, SC
12 December 2017